The Best Bay Area Restaurants for a Romantic Night Out

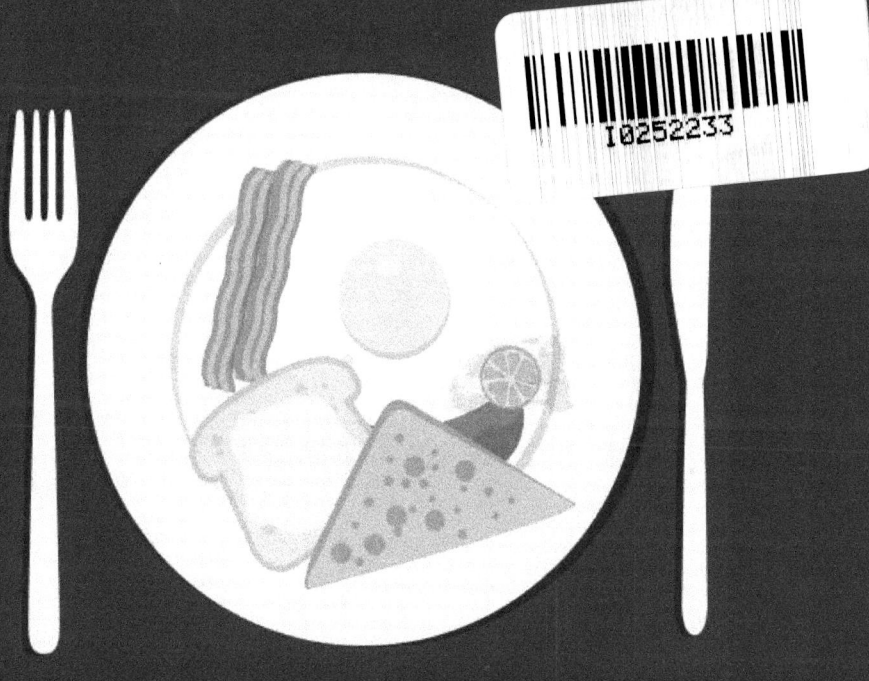

Kelly Anderson

The Best Bay Area Restaurants for a Romantic Night Out

Table Of Contents

Chapter 1: Introduction   3

   The Importance of Choosing the Right Restaurant   3

   What to Expect from This Guide   3

Chapter 2: The Bay Area Restaurant Scene   4

   San Francisco   4

   Oakland   5

   Berkeley   5

   San Jose   6

   Napa Valley   7

Chapter 3: Romantic Restaurants in the Bay Area   7

The Best Bay Area Restaurants for a Romantic Night Out

San Francisco	7
French Cuisine	8
Italian Cuisine	9
Seafood	9
Oakland	10
Farm-to-Table	11
Mexican Cuisine	12
Berkeley	12
Vegetarian and Vegan	13
Tapas	14
San Jose	14
Asian Cuisine	15

The Best Bay Area Restaurants for a Romantic Night Out

The Best Bay Area Restaurants for a Romantic Night Out

Steakhouse	16
Napa Valley	16
Wine Country Cuisine	17
Fine Dining	18
Chapter 4: Gluten-Free Dining in the Bay Area	**19**
San Francisco	19
Oakland	20
Berkeley	20
San Jose	21
Napa Valley	22
Chapter 5: Tips for Planning a Romantic Night Out	**22**
Making Reservations	22
Dress Code	23

The Best Bay Area Restaurants for a Romantic Night Out

    Transportation   24
    Preparing for Dietary Restrictions   24
Chapter 6: Conclusion   25
    Recap of Top Bay Area Romantic Restaurants   26
    Final Thoughts and Recommendations   26

The Best Bay Area Restaurants for a Romantic Night Out

Chapter 1: Introduction

The Importance of Choosing the Right Restaurant

When it comes to planning a romantic night out, choosing the right restaurant is key. The ambiance, food, and service can all make or break the experience. In the Bay Area, there are countless options for dining out, but not every restaurant is created equal. Here are a few reasons why choosing the right restaurant is so important.

First and foremost, the ambiance sets the tone for the evening. Whether you're looking for a cozy, intimate atmosphere or a more lively scene, the right restaurant can make all the difference. Think about the type of environment that will make you and your partner feel most comfortable and relaxed.

Of course, the food is also a crucial factor in choosing a restaurant. The Bay Area is known for its incredible culinary scene, so it's important to do your research and find a restaurant that specializes in the type of cuisine you're in the mood for. Whether you're in the mood for a classic steakhouse, fresh seafood, or innovative vegetarian dishes, there are plenty of options to choose from.

The Best Bay Area Restaurants for a Romantic Night Out

Another important consideration is service. A friendly and attentive staff can make the entire experience more enjoyable, while a rude or inattentive server can leave a bad taste in your mouth. Look for reviews online or ask friends for recommendations to find a restaurant with a reputation for excellent service.

For those with dietary restrictions, finding the right restaurant can be even more important. The Bay Area is home to a wide variety of gluten-free and other special diet-friendly restaurants, but it's important to do your research and make sure the restaurant you choose can accommodate your needs.

Overall, choosing the right restaurant is essential for a successful romantic night out. By considering factors like ambiance, food, service, and dietary restrictions, you can ensure that your evening is a memorable one.

What to Expect from This Guide

What to Expect from This Guide

Are you looking to treat your loved one to a romantic night out in the Bay Area? Look no further than "The Best Bay Area Restaurants for a Romantic Night Out." This guide is designed to help you find the perfect spot for a special evening with your partner.

For those with dietary restrictions, we also offer a Gluten-Free Bay Area Restaurant Guide, ensuring that everyone can indulge in a delicious meal without worry.

The Best Bay Area Restaurants for a Romantic Night Out

In this guide, we have carefully curated a list of the best restaurants in the Bay Area that offer romantic atmospheres, impeccable service, and delectable cuisine. From intimate, candlelit spaces to stunning waterfront views, we have something for every couple in search of a romantic evening.

We have also taken into consideration the varying price points of these restaurants, so whether you're on a tight budget or looking to splurge, we have options for everyone.

In addition to our restaurant recommendations, we also provide insider tips on how to make the most out of your romantic night out. From what to wear to how to plan the perfect surprise for your loved one, we've got you covered.

Overall, "The Best Bay Area Restaurants for a Romantic Night Out" and the Gluten-Free Bay Area Restaurant Guide are the ultimate resources for couples looking to have a memorable evening in the Bay Area. So sit back, relax, and let us guide you to the perfect spot for a romantic night out.

Chapter 2: The Bay Area Restaurant Scene

San Francisco

The Best Bay Area Restaurants for a Romantic Night Out

San Francisco is renowned for its diverse food scene, and it's no surprise that it's home to some of the best romantic restaurants in the Bay Area. Whether you're looking for a cozy spot for two or a fine dining experience, San Francisco has it all.

For those looking for a gluten-free option, Nourish Cafe is a must-visit. This plant-based cafe offers a variety of gluten-free options, including their famous gluten-free waffles. Their romantic atmosphere and delicious food make it the perfect place for a date night.

Another gluten-free option is Poesia. This Italian restaurant in the Castro offers a gluten-free menu that includes pasta dishes and pizza. The intimate ambiance and candlelit tables make it a perfect spot for a romantic night out.

For a fine dining experience, Quince is a must-visit. This Michelin-starred restaurant offers a tasting menu that features seasonal ingredients and Italian-inspired dishes. The elegant ambiance and impeccable service make it a perfect spot for a special occasion.

If you're looking for a cozy spot for two, Zuni Cafe is a great choice. This classic San Francisco restaurant offers a warm and inviting atmosphere, with a menu that features local and seasonal ingredients. Their famous roast chicken for two is a must-try, and the romantic ambiance makes it a perfect spot for a date night.

The Best Bay Area Restaurants for a Romantic Night Out

For those looking for a unique dining experience, Foreign Cinema is a must-visit. This restaurant offers a variety of global-inspired dishes, and their outdoor courtyard is transformed into a movie theater at night. The romantic setting and delicious food make it a perfect spot for a memorable night out.

In conclusion, San Francisco offers a diverse range of romantic restaurants, making it the perfect destination for a night out with your significant other. From cozy spots for two to fine dining experiences, San Francisco has something for everyone. And with gluten-free options available at many restaurants, those with dietary restrictions can still enjoy a romantic night out in the Bay Area.

Oakland

Oakland is a vibrant and diverse city that offers some of the best restaurants in the Bay Area. Whether you're looking for a romantic night out or just a delicious meal, Oakland has something for everyone.

For those who are gluten-free, Oakland has plenty of options. One of the best restaurants in town is Homeroom, which specializes in mac and cheese. They offer several gluten-free options, including a gluten-free mac and cheese that is to die for. Another great option is Nido Kitchen and Bar, which serves up delicious Mexican cuisine with plenty of gluten-free options.

The Best Bay Area Restaurants for a Romantic Night Out

If you're looking for a romantic night out, look no further than Commis. This Michelin-starred restaurant offers a prix-fixe menu that changes frequently, featuring seasonal ingredients and innovative dishes. The intimate setting and impeccable service make it the perfect spot for a special occasion.

For a more casual date night, head to The Wolf. This cozy restaurant serves up delicious comfort food, with a focus on locally-sourced ingredients. Their menu changes frequently, but you can always expect hearty dishes like fried chicken and biscuits, or a hearty bowl of pasta.

Another great option for a romantic night out is Lake Chalet. This waterfront restaurant offers stunning views of Lake Merritt, and their menu focuses on locally-sourced seafood. They offer several gluten-free options, including a delicious seafood stew that is perfect for sharing.

No matter what type of cuisine you're in the mood for, Oakland has something for everyone. From cozy comfort food to Michelin-starred fine dining, you're sure to find the perfect spot for a romantic night out.

Berkeley

Berkeley

The Best Bay Area Restaurants for a Romantic Night Out

Berkeley is a city located in the East Bay region of the San Francisco Bay Area. It is famous for its vibrant food scene, which offers a diverse range of cuisines from around the world. Whether you're a foodie looking for the latest culinary trends or a couple looking for a romantic night out, Berkeley has something to offer.

One of the most popular restaurants in Berkeley is Chez Panisse. This iconic restaurant, founded by Alice Waters in 1971, is a pioneer of the farm-to-table movement. Chez Panisse offers a prix-fixe menu that changes daily based on the availability of local and seasonal ingredients. The restaurant's commitment to sustainability and local sourcing has earned it a reputation as one of the best restaurants in the world.

For those who prefer a more casual setting, Berkeley has plenty of options. The Cheese Board Collective is a popular spot for pizza lovers. This worker-owned cooperative offers vegetarian and vegan pizzas made with fresh, seasonal ingredients. The menu changes daily, so there's always something new to try.

If you're looking for a gluten-free option, head to Gather. This restaurant specializes in organic, locally sourced cuisine and offers a range of gluten-free dishes. The menu features seasonal vegetables, sustainably raised meats, and fresh seafood.

The Best Bay Area Restaurants for a Romantic Night Out

For a romantic night out, head to Comal. This upscale Mexican restaurant offers a cozy, candlelit atmosphere and a menu that highlights the bold flavors of regional Mexican cuisine. The restaurant's cocktail program is also top-notch, with a range of creative and well-crafted drinks to choose from.

Overall, Berkeley is a foodie's paradise, with something to offer for every palate and budget. From iconic restaurants to casual cafes, this city has it all. So, whether you're a local or just visiting, make sure to check out the best Bay Area restaurants for a romantic night out in Berkeley.

San Jose

San Jose is the third-largest city in California and boasts a diverse culinary scene that is sure to impress any foodie. From fine dining establishments to casual eateries, San Jose has something to offer everyone seeking a romantic night out. In this chapter, we will explore some of the best restaurants in San Jose that deliver an unforgettable dining experience.

One of the most popular restaurants in San Jose is Adega. This Michelin-starred restaurant serves Portuguese cuisine that is both authentic and innovative. The menu features dishes such as octopus carpaccio, roasted quail, and grilled sardines. Adega also offers an extensive wine list, with over 500 bottles to choose from. The restaurant's elegant decor and attentive service make it an ideal location for a romantic date night.

The Best Bay Area Restaurants for a Romantic Night Out

For those seeking a more casual dining experience, The Table is a must-visit restaurant in San Jose. This farm-to-table eatery sources its ingredients from local farmers and serves up dishes like roasted chicken, grilled salmon, and handmade pasta. The restaurant also has an extensive gluten-free menu, making it a perfect choice for those with dietary restrictions. The Table's cozy atmosphere and friendly staff make it a great option for a relaxed evening out.

Another standout restaurant in San Jose is Manresa. This three-Michelin-starred restaurant is located in nearby Los Gatos and delivers an exceptional dining experience. Chef David Kinch's menu features seasonal ingredients and showcases his unique culinary vision. Dishes like duck breast with huckleberries and roasted king salmon are sure to impress even the most discerning foodie. Manresa's elegant dining room and impeccable service make it an ideal location for a special occasion or romantic night out.

In conclusion, San Jose is a city that offers a diverse culinary landscape that is sure to satisfy any food lover. Whether you're seeking an upscale fine-dining experience or a more casual night out, San Jose has something to offer. Adega, The Table, and Manresa are just a few of the many exceptional restaurants that are worth a visit. So, if you're looking for a romantic night out in San Jose, be sure to check out these top-notch restaurants.

Napa Valley

The Best Bay Area Restaurants for a Romantic Night Out

Napa Valley is a world-renowned wine region located in the heart of California. It's a perfect destination for couples who love wine and want to experience the romantic atmosphere of the vineyards. Napa is known for its Michelin-starred restaurants, but it's also a great place for casual dining and exploring the local cuisine.

For a romantic night out, we recommend making reservations at Auberge du Soleil, one of the most famous restaurants in Napa Valley. This French-inspired restaurant boasts breathtaking views of the valley and offers a seasonal menu that highlights locally grown ingredients. Auberge du Soleil is a perfect spot for a special occasion or a romantic dinner for two.

Another great restaurant to visit in Napa Valley is The Restaurant at Meadowood. This Michelin-starred restaurant offers a unique dining experience by combining the beauty of the surrounding landscape with seasonal ingredients sourced from local farmers. The Restaurant at Meadowood is known for its inventive tasting menus and extensive wine list, making it a top choice for foodies and wine lovers alike.

If you're looking for a more casual dining experience, we recommend checking out Gott's Roadside. This popular burger joint offers a variety of burgers, salads, and sandwiches made with locally sourced, sustainable ingredients. Gott's Roadside also offers a great selection of wine and beer, making it a perfect spot for a casual date night.

The Best Bay Area Restaurants for a Romantic Night Out

For those with dietary restrictions, there are plenty of gluten-free options in Napa Valley. One of our top picks is Oxbow Public Market, a food hall that offers a variety of gluten-free options from local vendors. From fresh oysters to organic salads, Oxbow Public Market has something for everyone.

Overall, Napa Valley is a top destination for a romantic night out. With its breathtaking views, Michelin-starred restaurants, and locally sourced cuisine, it's no wonder why Napa is a favorite among foodies and wine lovers alike. Whether you're looking for a fancy dinner or a casual bite, Napa Valley has something for everyone.

Chapter 3: Romantic Restaurants in the Bay Area

San Francisco

San Francisco is a city that is known for its vibrant food scene. From the freshest seafood to the most innovative culinary creations, the city is a food lover's paradise. When it comes to planning a romantic night out in San Francisco, the options are endless. Here are some of the best restaurants in the city that are perfect for a romantic night out.

The Best Bay Area Restaurants for a Romantic Night Out

One of the most popular restaurants in San Francisco is Gary Danko. This is a perfect spot for those who are looking for a romantic and elegant dining experience. The restaurant offers a tasting menu that features dishes like lobster risotto, roasted duck breast, and chocolate souffle. The restaurant also has an extensive wine list that will complement your meal perfectly.

For those who are looking for an intimate and cozy dining experience, The Progress is a great option. The restaurant is located in the Mission District and offers a unique menu that is inspired by the flavors of California. The restaurant offers a family-style dining experience, which means that you will be able to share your meal with your loved one. The menu changes frequently, so make sure to check the restaurant's website before making a reservation.

If you are looking for a restaurant that offers gluten-free options, Coqueta is a great option. The restaurant is located on the Embarcadero and offers a menu that is inspired by the flavors of Spain. The restaurant offers a gluten-free menu that includes dishes like grilled octopus, roasted chicken, and paella. The restaurant also has a great selection of cocktails that are perfect for a romantic night out.

Another great option for those who are looking for a gluten-free restaurant is Nopa. The restaurant is located in the Western Addition and offers a menu that is inspired by the flavors of California. The restaurant offers a gluten-free menu that includes dishes like grilled pork chops, roasted salmon, and quinoa salad. The restaurant also has a great selection of wines that will complement your meal perfectly.

The Best Bay Area Restaurants for a Romantic Night Out

In conclusion, San Francisco is a city that offers a wide range of dining options for those who are looking for a romantic night out. Whether you are looking for an elegant and upscale dining experience or a cozy and intimate spot, there is something for everyone in this vibrant city. Make sure to check out these restaurants the next time you are planning a romantic night out in San Francisco.

French Cuisine

French Cuisine

When it comes to romantic dining, few cuisines are as celebrated as French cuisine. With its rich flavors, classic dishes, and elegant presentation, French food has been a favorite of foodies and romantics for centuries. Fortunately, the Bay Area is home to some of the best French restaurants in the country, offering a taste of Paris right here in California.

One of the most popular French restaurants in the Bay Area is La Folie, located in San Francisco's Russian Hill neighborhood. This Michelin-starred restaurant is known for its exquisite tasting menus, which showcase the best of French cuisine with a modern twist. Dishes like foie gras torchon, lobster bisque, and roasted duck breast are expertly prepared and presented, making for an unforgettable dining experience.

The Best Bay Area Restaurants for a Romantic Night Out

Another beloved French restaurant in the Bay Area is Chez Panisse, located in Berkeley. This iconic establishment was founded by chef Alice Waters in 1971 and has since become a symbol of the farm-to-table movement. The menu changes daily depending on what's fresh and in season, but you can always expect dishes like roasted chicken, grilled fish, and colorful vegetable platters that celebrate the bounty of the Bay Area.

For a more casual French dining experience, head to Bistro Jeanty in Yountville. This cozy bistro serves up classic French comfort food like onion soup, escargots, and steak frites, all in a charming, rustic atmosphere. The wine list is extensive and features many local Napa Valley wines, making it the perfect spot for a romantic date night.

If you're looking for a French restaurant with gluten-free options, check out Café Claude in San Francisco. This cozy bistro offers a variety of gluten-free dishes, including steak tartare, mussels, and roasted chicken, all of which are prepared with the same care and attention to detail as their regular menu items.

Whether you're a die-hard Francophile or just looking for a special date night spot, the Bay Area's French restaurants are sure to satisfy. From refined tasting menus to rustic bistro fare, there's something for everyone in this culinary capital of the West Coast.

Italian Cuisine

Italian Cuisine

The Best Bay Area Restaurants for a Romantic Night Out

Italian cuisine is one of the most popular cuisines in the world. It is famous for its simple yet delicious flavors. Italian cuisine is all about using fresh ingredients and letting the natural flavors shine through. The Bay Area has some of the best Italian restaurants in the world, and it is the perfect place to enjoy a romantic night out.

Italian cuisine is known for its wide variety of pasta dishes. The most popular pasta dishes include spaghetti, lasagna, penne, and fettuccine. Italian restaurants in the Bay Area usually make their pasta from scratch, giving it a unique texture and taste. If you are gluten-free, many Italian restaurants offer gluten-free pasta options.

Apart from pasta, Italian cuisine is also famous for its pizza. The Bay Area has some of the best pizza places in the world, serving authentic Neapolitan-style pizza. The pizza is made using fresh ingredients, including San Marzano tomatoes, mozzarella cheese, and fresh basil.

Italian cuisine also includes a variety of meat and seafood dishes. Some of the popular meat dishes include Osso Buco, Veal Scallopini, and Chicken Parmigiana. Seafood lovers can enjoy dishes like Linguine with Clams, Calamari Fritti, and Grilled Octopus.

No Italian meal is complete without a glass of wine. The Bay Area has some of the best wine regions in the world, and Italian restaurants offer an extensive selection of Italian wines. You can enjoy a glass of Chianti or Barolo with your meal to enhance the flavors of your dish.

The Best Bay Area Restaurants for a Romantic Night Out

In conclusion, Italian cuisine is the perfect choice for a romantic night out in the Bay Area. Italian restaurants in the Bay Area offer a wide variety of dishes, including pasta, pizza, meat, and seafood dishes. If you are gluten-free, many Italian restaurants offer gluten-free pasta options. You can also enjoy a glass of Italian wine to complete your meal.

Seafood

Seafood is a popular cuisine in the Bay Area, thanks to the region's proximity to the Pacific Ocean. From Dungeness crab to oysters, the Bay Area is home to a wide variety of seafood options that are perfect for a romantic night out. In this subchapter, we will explore some of the best seafood restaurants in the Bay Area that cater to both the bay area restaurant guide and Gluten-Free Bay Area Restaurant Guide niches.

One of the top seafood restaurants in the Bay Area is Waterbar. Located in San Francisco, Waterbar offers stunning views of the Bay and the Bay Bridge. Their menu focuses on sustainable seafood, including Dungeness crab, oysters, and a variety of fish. For those looking for gluten-free options, Waterbar offers gluten-free bread and several gluten-free dishes, including the Grilled Fish Tacos and the Crispy Skin Salmon.

Another great seafood restaurant in the Bay Area is the Fish Market in San Mateo. This restaurant has been serving fresh seafood since 1976 and is known for its seafood chowder and cioppino. For those with gluten sensitivities, the Fish Market has a separate gluten-free menu that includes dishes like the Grilled Salmon and the Jumbo Prawn Cocktail.

The Best Bay Area Restaurants for a Romantic Night Out

For a more intimate dining experience, head to La Ciccia in San Francisco. This cozy Italian restaurant specializes in Sardinian cuisine and features a variety of seafood dishes, including the Grilled Octopus and the Spaghetti with Bottarga. La Ciccia also offers gluten-free pasta options, making it a great choice for those following a gluten-free diet.

If you're in the mood for sushi, head to Tataki in San Francisco. This sustainable sushi restaurant offers a variety of gluten-free options, including the Wild Salmon Sashimi and the Grilled Shishito Peppers. Tataki also has a strict no-tipping policy and donates a portion of their profits to environmental causes.

In conclusion, the Bay Area is home to some of the best seafood restaurants in the country. Whether you're looking for sustainable seafood, gluten-free options, or an intimate dining experience, there's a seafood restaurant in the Bay Area that will meet your needs.

Oakland

Oakland is a city full of culture, diversity, and vibrant energy. It's no surprise that this city also boasts some of the best restaurants in the Bay Area. Whether you're looking for a romantic night out or just a delicious meal, Oakland has something for everyone.

The Best Bay Area Restaurants for a Romantic Night Out

One of the top restaurants in Oakland is Commis, a Michelin-starred restaurant that offers a tasting menu of contemporary Californian cuisine. The menu changes frequently, but expect dishes like smoked sturgeon with caviar, beef tartare with burnt onion, and roasted duck with persimmon. Commis is an ideal spot for a special occasion or a romantic night out.

Another top restaurant in Oakland is Homestead, which is known for its farm-to-table cuisine and cozy atmosphere. The menu changes seasonally, but expect dishes like wood-grilled octopus, crispy pork belly, and roasted chicken with lemon and thyme. Homestead also offers an extensive wine list, making it a perfect spot for a romantic dinner for two.

For those in search of gluten-free options, The Kebabery is a great choice. This Mediterranean-style restaurant offers a variety of kebabs, salads, and sides, all of which are gluten-free. The lamb kebab with cucumber yogurt and the spiced chicken kebab with harissa are both delicious choices. The Kebabery also offers vegetarian and vegan options, making it a great spot for groups with different dietary needs.

If you're in the mood for seafood, Reem's California is the perfect spot. This Lebanese-inspired restaurant offers a variety of seafood dishes, including grilled shrimp with garlic and lemon, seared salmon with tahini sauce, and crispy fried whole fish. Reem's California also offers a variety of vegetarian and gluten-free options, making it a great spot for groups with different dietary needs.

The Best Bay Area Restaurants for a Romantic Night Out

Oakland is a city full of hidden gems, and these restaurants are just a few of the many great options available. Whether you're looking for a romantic night out or just a delicious meal, Oakland has something for everyone.

Farm-to-Table

Farm-to-Table

Farm-to-table is a term used to describe the process of sourcing ingredients directly from local farms and serving them fresh at the table. The Bay Area is known for its abundance of small, family-owned farms and organic produce, making it the perfect destination for farm-to-table dining experiences.

At the heart of farm-to-table dining is the concept of sustainability. By sourcing ingredients locally, restaurants can reduce their carbon footprint by eliminating the need for long-distance transportation. Furthermore, buying from small-scale farmers supports the local economy and promotes sustainable agriculture practices.

Many Bay Area restaurants have embraced the farm-to-table concept and have made it a core part of their culinary philosophy. Some of the best restaurants in the area, such as Chez Panisse and The French Laundry, have been pioneers in the farm-to-table movement, and have set the standard for others to follow.

The Best Bay Area Restaurants for a Romantic Night Out

Farm-to-table dining is not just about the ingredients, but also about the experience. Many restaurants in the Bay Area have created beautiful outdoor dining spaces that allow diners to connect with nature while enjoying their meals. These spaces often feature gardens and outdoor seating areas that provide a unique ambiance and enhance the overall dining experience.

For those with dietary restrictions, farm-to-table dining can be a great option. Many Bay Area restaurants offer gluten-free options, and with the use of fresh, locally sourced ingredients, it can be easier to find dishes that are free of allergens and artificial additives.

Overall, farm-to-table dining is a unique and enjoyable experience that allows diners to connect with their food and the local community. Whether you're a foodie looking for the latest culinary trends or a health-conscious individual looking for fresh, wholesome meals, the Bay Area's farm-to-table restaurants have something to offer everyone.

Mexican Cuisine

Mexican Cuisine

Mexican cuisine is a favorite among many people, and the Bay Area has some of the best Mexican restaurants around. From traditional dishes to modern interpretations, there is something for everyone.

The Best Bay Area Restaurants for a Romantic Night Out

One of the best places to experience authentic Mexican cuisine is at La Taqueria in San Francisco. They are known for their delicious tacos, made with freshly cooked meats and homemade tortillas. The atmosphere is casual, but the food is top-notch.

If you're looking for a more upscale experience, head over to Calavera in Oakland. This restaurant offers a modern take on Mexican cuisine, with dishes like octopus ceviche and roasted pork shoulder. The decor is stylish and modern, making it a great spot for a romantic night out.

For those who are gluten-free, Nopalito in San Francisco is a great option. They offer a wide variety of gluten-free options, including their famous guacamole and mole. The restaurant has a warm and inviting atmosphere, making it a great place for a date night.

Another great restaurant for gluten-free options is Tacolicious in San Francisco. They offer a variety of gluten-free tacos, including their popular Baja-style fish taco. The atmosphere is lively and fun, making it a great spot for a night out with friends.

No matter what type of Mexican cuisine you're in the mood for, the Bay Area has something to offer. From traditional to modern, casual to upscale, there is a restaurant to fit every taste and budget. So, grab some friends or your significant other and head out to explore the delicious flavors of Mexican cuisine in the Bay Area.

Berkeley

The Best Bay Area Restaurants for a Romantic Night Out

Berkeley is a city well-known for its vibrant foodie scene. The city is home to various restaurants that cater to different dietary restrictions, including gluten-free options. Whether you're looking for a romantic dinner with your significant other or a group gathering with friends, Berkeley has a restaurant to suit your needs.

One of the most popular restaurants in Berkeley is Chez Panisse. The restaurant is famous for its farm-to-table cuisine that highlights locally-sourced ingredients. The menu changes seasonally to ensure that only the freshest ingredients are used. Chez Panisse offers a romantic and intimate atmosphere that is perfect for a special night out.

Another great restaurant in Berkeley is Gather. The restaurant is known for its delicious vegetarian and vegan options. Gather's menu is seasonal and features ingredients from local farmers and artisans. The ambiance is warm and cozy, making it a great spot for a romantic date.

If you're in the mood for Italian cuisine, head to Trattoria Corso. The restaurant offers a menu that is both gluten-free and vegetarian-friendly. The ambiance is casual and laid-back, making it a great spot for a low-key night out.

For a unique dining experience, head to Comal. The restaurant offers a modern take on Mexican cuisine and features a menu that is both gluten-free and vegetarian-friendly. Comal's atmosphere is lively and energetic, making it a great spot for a group gathering with friends.

The Best Bay Area Restaurants for a Romantic Night Out

Berkeley is a city that offers a diverse range of dining options. Whether you're looking for a romantic night out or a group gathering with friends, there is a restaurant in Berkeley to suit your needs. With its farm-to-table cuisine, vegan and gluten-free options, and unique dining experiences, Berkeley is a must-visit destination for foodies in the Bay Area.

Vegetarian and Vegan

Vegetarian and Vegan

For those who prefer a plant-based diet, the Bay Area has plenty of options for a romantic night out. Whether you are a strict vegan or a flexitarian looking for meat-free meals, the following restaurants offer creative and delicious vegetarian and vegan options that will satisfy your appetite and impress your date.

Gracias Madre

Located in the Mission District of San Francisco, Gracias Madre is a vegan Mexican restaurant that serves organic and locally sourced ingredients. The menu features a variety of plant-based dishes such as the jackfruit carnitas tacos, the mole enchiladas, and the coconut ceviche. The restaurant also offers a selection of vegan cocktails, wines, and beers to complement your meal.

Millennium

The Best Bay Area Restaurants for a Romantic Night Out

As one of the most famous vegetarian restaurants in the Bay Area, Millennium is a must-visit destination for veggie lovers. Located in Oakland, this upscale restaurant offers a diverse menu of creative and flavorful dishes that showcase seasonal and organic produce. The menu changes frequently, but some of the popular items include the wild mushroom risotto, the grilled seitan skewers, and the coconut curry noodles.

Shizen Vegan Sushi Bar & Izakaya

If you are a sushi lover, but don't eat fish, Shizen Vegan Sushi Bar & Izakaya is the perfect spot for you. Located in the Mission District of San Francisco, this vegan sushi bar offers a wide range of plant-based sushi rolls and izakaya-style dishes such as the crispy brussels sprouts, the karaage chicken, and the spicy miso ramen. The restaurant also has a selection of sake, beer, and cocktails to accompany your meal.

The Plant Cafe Organic

With multiple locations in San Francisco and the Bay Area, The Plant Cafe Organic is a casual yet elegant restaurant that serves healthy and sustainable food. The menu features a variety of vegetarian and vegan options such as the plant-based burger, the quinoa bowl, and the roasted cauliflower steak. The restaurant also offers a selection of organic wines, beers, and juices to complement your meal.

The Best Bay Area Restaurants for a Romantic Night Out

In conclusion, the Bay Area has a rich and diverse culinary scene that caters to different dietary needs and preferences. Whether you are a vegetarian, vegan, or simply looking for meat-free options, these restaurants offer some of the best plant-based meals in the area. So, why not surprise your date with a romantic night out at one of these veggie-friendly spots?

Tapas

Tapas

If you're looking for a romantic night out at a Bay Area restaurant, you can't go wrong with tapas. These small plates are perfect for sharing, and they allow you to try a variety of different dishes without committing to a full-sized entrée.

One of the best places to try tapas in the Bay Area is at Canela Bistro & Wine Bar in San Francisco. This cozy restaurant offers a wide range of Spanish-inspired dishes, from patatas bravas to grilled octopus to chorizo-stuffed dates. And if you're gluten-free, they have plenty of options for you too, like their crispy eggplant with romesco sauce or their shrimp and avocado salad.

The Best Bay Area Restaurants for a Romantic Night Out

Another great spot for tapas is Teleferic Barcelona in Walnut Creek and Palo Alto. This stylish restaurant serves up classic Spanish dishes like tortilla española and jamón ibérico, as well as more modern creations like their squid ink paella and their "patatas bravas 2.0" with spicy tomato foam. And if you're gluten-free, they have a dedicated menu with options like their grilled octopus with romesco sauce or their sautéed mushrooms with garlic and parsley.

For a more upscale tapas experience, head to Coqueta on the Embarcadero in San Francisco. This Michelin-starred restaurant offers stunning views of the Bay Bridge and a menu that highlights the best of Spanish cuisine. Try their crispy pork belly with quince purée, their grilled octopus with fingerling potatoes, or their chorizo and potato bombas. And if you're gluten-free, they have plenty of options for you too, like their gambas al ajillo (garlic shrimp) or their wood-grilled beef skewers with romesco sauce.

No matter where you go for tapas in the Bay Area, you're sure to have a romantic and delicious night out. So grab your partner and get ready to share some small plates and some big love.

San Jose

San Jose is a bustling city located in the heart of the Silicon Valley. It is the third-largest city in California and is home to a diverse community that has contributed to the city's vibrant food scene. San Jose has a wide range of restaurants that cater to all tastes and preferences, making it an excellent destination for a romantic night out.

The Best Bay Area Restaurants for a Romantic Night Out

If you're looking for a romantic night out, San Jose has plenty of options to choose from. One restaurant that stands out is the Adega, a Michelin-starred Portuguese restaurant that offers a contemporary twist on traditional Portuguese cuisine. The restaurant's elegant decor and intimate atmosphere make it the perfect place for a romantic dinner. You can indulge in their seafood dishes, such as garlic shrimp or octopus, or try their famous suckling pig.

For those who are gluten-free, Dio Deka is the perfect choice. This Mediterranean restaurant offers a gluten-free menu that includes a variety of dishes, such as grilled lamb chops and roasted beet salad. The restaurant has a cozy and intimate atmosphere that is perfect for a romantic night out. The restaurant also has an extensive wine list that includes many local and international selections.

Another option for a romantic night out is The Table. This restaurant offers a farm-to-table dining experience that emphasizes locally sourced ingredients. They have a seasonal menu that changes frequently to ensure that you get the freshest ingredients. The restaurant's cozy and intimate atmosphere makes it a perfect choice for a romantic dinner. They also have an extensive wine list that includes many local and international selections.

In conclusion, San Jose is a great destination for a romantic night out. The city offers a diverse range of restaurants that cater to all tastes and preferences. Whether you're looking for a Michelin-starred restaurant or a cozy farm-to-table dining experience, San Jose has something to offer. So, why not book a table at one of these amazing restaurants and enjoy a romantic night out in San Jose?

The Best Bay Area Restaurants for a Romantic Night Out

Asian Cuisine

Asian Cuisine

The Bay Area is well-known for its diverse culinary offerings, and Asian cuisine is no exception. From sushi to dim sum, there are countless options for those looking to indulge in the flavors of the Far East. Whether you're looking for a romantic night out or simply searching for some delicious gluten-free options, the Bay Area has plenty to offer.

One of the most popular Asian cuisines in the Bay Area is Japanese. Sushi lovers will be delighted by the many options available, from traditional nigiri to creative rolls with unique flavor combinations. For an upscale experience, check out Akiko's Restaurant in San Francisco, which offers a variety of fresh and innovative sushi dishes. Another great option is ICHI Sushi in Oakland, which features sustainably-sourced ingredients and a cozy, intimate setting.

For those who prefer Chinese cuisine, dim sum is a must-try. This Cantonese tradition involves small, bite-sized dishes served on small plates or in steamer baskets. Yank Sing in San Francisco is a popular spot for dim sum, offering a wide variety of options including vegetarian and gluten-free dishes. Koi Palace in Daly City is another top-rated dim sum destination, known for its extensive menu and beautiful decor.

The Best Bay Area Restaurants for a Romantic Night Out

Thai cuisine is also popular in the Bay Area, with its bold flavors and fresh ingredients. One standout restaurant is Farmhouse Kitchen Thai Cuisine in Oakland, which offers an extensive gluten-free menu and a cozy, rustic atmosphere. Another great option is Kin Khao in San Francisco, which features modern Thai cuisine with a focus on locally-sourced ingredients.

Whether you're looking for a romantic night out or simply searching for some delicious gluten-free options, the Bay Area's Asian cuisine has something for everyone. From sushi to dim sum to Thai curries, there are countless options to explore and enjoy.

Steakhouse

The Bay Area is home to some of the best steakhouses in the country. Whether you're celebrating a special occasion or just looking for a romantic night out, these restaurants are sure to impress.

One of the top steakhouses in the Bay Area is Alexander's Steakhouse. This upscale restaurant offers a modern twist on the classic steakhouse experience, with innovative dishes like wagyu beef sushi and foie gras sliders. The restaurant also boasts an extensive wine list, making it the perfect spot for a special occasion.

The Best Bay Area Restaurants for a Romantic Night Out

For those looking for a more traditional steakhouse experience, there's Harris' Restaurant in San Francisco. This family-owned restaurant has been serving up classic steaks since 1984. The menu features USDA Prime beef, dry-aged in-house, and cooked to perfection over an open flame. The restaurant also has an impressive selection of vintage wines and rare spirits.

If you're looking for a steakhouse that caters to gluten-free diners, look no further than Boboquivari's in San Francisco. This classic steakhouse offers a wide variety of gluten-free options, from the filet mignon to the lobster tail. The restaurant also has an extensive wine list and a cozy, intimate atmosphere that's perfect for a romantic night out.

No matter which steakhouse you choose, you're sure to have a memorable dining experience in the Bay Area. From modern twists on classic dishes to traditional steakhouses with a rich history, there's something for everyone in this restaurant-rich region.

Napa Valley

Napa Valley is a world-renowned viticultural region located just an hour's drive from San Francisco. This picturesque valley is home to some of the best wineries, Michelin-starred restaurants, and breathtaking views. The perfect place for a romantic night out, Napa Valley offers an unforgettable experience that will leave you wanting more.

The Best Bay Area Restaurants for a Romantic Night Out

For the gluten-free bay area restaurant guide, Napa Valley has plenty of options that cater to dietary restrictions. From the French Laundry to the Farmstead at Long Meadow Ranch, there are many restaurants that offer gluten-free menus. The French Laundry, located in Yountville, is a three-Michelin-starred restaurant that offers an exceptional dining experience. The restaurant's menu changes daily, but gluten-free options are always available. Farmstead at Long Meadow Ranch is another great option that offers gluten-free dishes made with locally sourced ingredients.

For those looking for a more intimate setting, Auberge du Soleil is a must-visit. This Michelin-starred restaurant offers panoramic views of Napa Valley and a menu that focuses on locally sourced ingredients. The restaurant's menu changes seasonally, but there are always gluten-free options available.

If you're looking for something a little more casual, Gott's Roadside is the perfect spot. This popular burger joint offers gluten-free buns and a wide variety of toppings to choose from. Located in St. Helena, Gott's Roadside is a great place to stop for lunch or dinner while exploring Napa Valley.

Aside from the food, Napa Valley is also known for its incredible wineries. From the famous Napa Valley Wine Train to the countless vineyards that dot the valley, there is no shortage of options for wine lovers. Take a tour of some of the region's most famous wineries, such as Opus One or Sterling Vineyards, and enjoy a tasting of some of the world's best wines.

The Best Bay Area Restaurants for a Romantic Night Out

In conclusion, Napa Valley is a must-visit destination for anyone looking for a romantic night out. Whether you're looking for a Michelin-starred restaurant or a casual burger joint, there are plenty of options that cater to both gluten-free and non-gluten-free diners. With breathtaking views, world-class wineries, and exceptional dining experiences, Napa Valley is sure to leave you with memories that will last a lifetime.

Wine Country Cuisine

Wine Country Cuisine

The Bay Area is renowned for its wine country, and with that comes a unique style of cuisine. Wine country cuisine is all about pairing the right wine with the right dish, and the Bay Area has some of the best wine country cuisine restaurants in the country.

One of the best things about wine country cuisine is the focus on fresh, seasonal ingredients. Many of the restaurants in the Bay Area source their ingredients locally, which ensures that the food is not only delicious but also sustainable.

If you're looking for a romantic night out, why not try one of the many wine country cuisine restaurants in the Bay Area? Here are some of the best:

1. The French Laundry - This iconic restaurant in Yountville is known for its impeccable service and exquisite tasting menu. The restaurant is located in a beautiful old stone building, and the garden outside provides many of the ingredients for the dishes.

The Best Bay Area Restaurants for a Romantic Night Out

2. Farmstead at Long Meadow Ranch - Located in St. Helena, this restaurant is all about farm-to-table cuisine. The menu changes seasonally, but you can always expect fresh, locally sourced ingredients. The outdoor patio is perfect for a romantic dinner under the stars.

3. The Girl and the Fig - This restaurant in Sonoma is a must-visit for anyone who loves French cuisine. The focus is on seasonal ingredients, and the menu includes classic dishes like coq au vin and steak frites. The cozy atmosphere is perfect for a romantic night out.

If you're looking for a gluten-free option, there are plenty of wine country cuisine restaurants in the Bay Area that cater to those with dietary restrictions. Here are some of the best gluten-free restaurants in wine country:

1. Press - This restaurant in St. Helena has a separate gluten-free menu that includes dishes like crispy pork belly and grilled lamb chops. The atmosphere is upscale, but the staff is friendly and accommodating.

2. Bottega - This Italian restaurant in Yountville has a gluten-free menu that includes homemade pasta dishes and wood-fired pizzas. The restaurant is located in a beautiful old building, and the outdoor patio is perfect for a romantic dinner.

3. Poggio Trattoria - This Italian restaurant in Sausalito has a separate gluten-free menu that includes dishes like risotto and grilled fish. The restaurant is located right on the water, and the views are stunning.

The Best Bay Area Restaurants for a Romantic Night Out

No matter what your dietary restrictions are, there's a wine country cuisine restaurant in the Bay Area that's perfect for a romantic night out. So why not try one tonight?

Fine Dining

Fine Dining

For those who are looking for a romantic night out with their special someone, fine dining restaurants in the Bay Area are the perfect choice. These restaurants offer a unique dining experience that is unparalleled in terms of quality, presentation, and service. The Bay Area has a variety of fine dining restaurants that cater to different tastes and preferences. From French cuisine to American, Italian, and Asian, there is something for everyone.

One of the top fine dining restaurants in the Bay Area is the renowned Gary Danko restaurant. Located in San Francisco, Gary Danko is known for its elegant atmosphere, impeccable service, and an extensive menu of contemporary American and French cuisine. The restaurant offers a prix-fixe menu that changes daily, featuring seasonal ingredients and creative culinary techniques.

The Best Bay Area Restaurants for a Romantic Night Out

For those with dietary restrictions, the Bay Area has a variety of gluten-free fine dining restaurants that cater to their needs. One such restaurant is the popular Coi, located in San Francisco. Coi offers a tasting menu that features organic, locally-sourced ingredients with an emphasis on seafood. The restaurant also offers a gluten-free tasting menu that is specially prepared for guests with dietary restrictions.

Another fine dining restaurant that caters to the gluten-free niche is Madera, located in Menlo Park. Madera offers a farm-to-table menu, featuring organic and sustainably-raised ingredients. The restaurant has a separate gluten-free menu that includes a variety of dishes such as grilled octopus, roasted beet salad, and pan-seared scallops.

Fine dining restaurants in the Bay Area are not just about the food; they are also about the ambiance and atmosphere. These restaurants offer a romantic setting that is perfect for a special occasion or a date night. The decor is elegant, the lighting is dim, and the music is soothing, creating a romantic atmosphere that is perfect for couples.

In conclusion, the Bay Area is home to some of the best fine dining restaurants in the country. From the elegant Gary Danko to the gluten-free Coi and Madera, there is something for everyone. Whether you are looking for a romantic setting, impeccable service, or creative culinary techniques, the Bay Area has it all. So, if you are looking for a memorable night out with your special someone, consider one of these fine dining restaurants and experience the best of Bay Area cuisine.

# Chapter 4: Gluten-Free Dining in the Bay Area

San Francisco

San Francisco, known for its iconic Golden Gate Bridge, cable cars, and diverse culture, is also home to some of the best restaurants in the Bay Area. Whether you're looking for a cozy spot for a romantic dinner or a trendy spot for a night out with friends, San Francisco has something for everyone.

One restaurant that stands out is Gary Danko, located in the Fisherman's Wharf area. Chef Gary Danko offers a multi-course tasting menu that features seasonal ingredients and unique flavor combinations. The restaurant's elegant atmosphere and impeccable service make it a perfect choice for a special occasion or romantic night out.

For those following a gluten-free diet, Nopa in the Hayes Valley neighborhood is a great option. The restaurant's menu features a variety of gluten-free options, including a delicious roasted chicken dish with seasonal vegetables. The lively atmosphere and communal seating make for a fun and casual night out.

The Best Bay Area Restaurants for a Romantic Night Out

If you're in the mood for Italian cuisine, head to Cotogna in the Financial District. The restaurant's rustic decor and cozy ambiance make for a romantic setting. The menu features house-made pasta dishes and wood-fired pizzas, all made with locally sourced ingredients.

For a unique dining experience, check out The Progress in the Fillmore neighborhood. The restaurant offers a family-style menu that changes frequently, featuring dishes inspired by global flavors and techniques. The communal seating and lively atmosphere make for a fun and memorable night out with friends.

San Francisco is also home to a thriving cocktail scene, with many restaurants offering creative and innovative drinks. The Slanted Door in the Ferry Building is known for its Asian-inspired cocktails, while Trick Dog in the Mission District offers playful and whimsical drinks.

No matter what type of cuisine or atmosphere you're looking for, San Francisco has plenty of options for a romantic night out or a fun night with friends.

Oakland

Oakland is a vibrant city with a diverse culinary scene that has something for everyone. Whether you are looking for a romantic dinner with your significant other or a fun night out with friends, Oakland has plenty of options to satisfy your appetite.

The Best Bay Area Restaurants for a Romantic Night Out

If you are a fan of Italian cuisine, then you should check out Pizzaiolo. This restaurant offers a cozy atmosphere and serves up delicious wood-fired pizzas that are made with local and seasonal ingredients. They also have an extensive wine list that pairs perfectly with their dishes.

For a more upscale dining experience, Commis is a Michelin-starred restaurant that offers a tasting menu that changes seasonally. Their dishes are beautifully presented and incorporate unique flavors and textures that will leave a lasting impression on your taste buds.

If you are a gluten-free diner, then Homestead is the perfect spot for you. This farm-to-table restaurant offers a menu that is entirely gluten-free and features dishes that are made with locally sourced ingredients. Their cozy atmosphere and friendly staff make it the perfect place for a romantic night out.

For a more casual dining experience, head over to Hawker Fare. This Southeast Asian street food restaurant offers a lively atmosphere and serves up delicious dishes like crispy pork belly and chicken wings. They also have an extensive beer and cocktail menu that will keep you coming back for more.

No matter what your culinary preferences are, Oakland has plenty of options to choose from. Whether you are looking for a romantic night out or a fun night out with friends, you are sure to find something that will satisfy your appetite. So, be sure to check out these restaurants and explore all that Oakland has to offer.

The Best Bay Area Restaurants for a Romantic Night Out

Berkeley

Berkeley is a vibrant city located just across the bay from San Francisco, known for its charming tree-lined streets, diverse culture, and thriving food scene. For those looking for a romantic night out, Berkeley has no shortage of exceptional restaurants to choose from.

One of the top picks for a romantic evening in Berkeley is Chez Panisse. This renowned restaurant, founded by Alice Waters in 1971, is a pioneer of the farm-to-table movement and has been consistently recognized as one of the best restaurants in the country. The menu changes daily, featuring fresh and seasonal ingredients sourced from local farms and purveyors. The intimate dining room and attentive service make for a truly special experience.

For those with dietary restrictions, Gather is a must-try. This innovative restaurant offers a creative vegetarian and vegan menu, with many gluten-free options available. The sleek and modern space, complete with a rooftop garden, is the perfect backdrop for a romantic evening. The craft cocktails and extensive wine list are also not to be missed.

Another standout in Berkeley is Comal. This Mexican-inspired restaurant serves up delicious and authentic dishes made with locally-sourced ingredients. The warm and inviting atmosphere, complete with a cozy fireplace, is perfect for a romantic night out. The tequila and mezcal selection is also impressive, making for a fun and festive evening.

The Best Bay Area Restaurants for a Romantic Night Out

For a unique and unforgettable dining experience, head to the Gaumenkitzel German restaurant. This cozy and charming spot serves up classic German dishes made with organic and sustainable ingredients. The menu includes many gluten-free options, making it a great choice for those with dietary restrictions. The intimate atmosphere and attentive service make for a memorable evening.

Whether you're looking for a classic fine dining experience or something more casual and creative, Berkeley has something for everyone. With its dynamic food scene and charming ambiance, it's no wonder that Berkeley has become a favorite destination for food lovers and romantics alike.

San Jose

San Jose is one of the most vibrant cities in the Bay Area, offering a diverse selection of restaurants that cater to every palate. Whether you're looking for a romantic evening with your significant other or simply a night out with friends, San Jose has something to offer.

For those seeking a gluten-free dining experience, there are several restaurants in San Jose that cater to this dietary restriction. One such restaurant is The Table, which offers a gluten-free menu that includes dishes such as the grilled octopus with roasted fingerling potatoes and the pan-seared salmon with a citrus vinaigrette. Another great option is the Michelin-starred Adega Restaurant, which offers a gluten-free tasting menu that highlights the flavors of Portugal.

The Best Bay Area Restaurants for a Romantic Night Out

If you're in the mood for Italian cuisine, Il Fornaio is a must-visit restaurant in San Jose. The menu features classic Italian dishes such as pasta alla carbonara and osso buco, as well as gluten-free options such as the gluten-free pizza with prosciutto and arugula.

For a more upscale dining experience, The Plumed Horse is the perfect choice. This Michelin-starred restaurant offers a tasting menu that changes seasonally, featuring dishes such as the roasted duck breast with spiced quince and the sea scallops with cauliflower puree.

If you're looking for a more casual dining experience, San Jose also offers a variety of options. For a unique twist on Mexican cuisine, check out Luna Mexican Kitchen, which offers dishes such as the pork belly tacos and the chile relleno with quinoa and black beans. For a taste of Japan, head to Gombei Japanese Restaurant, which offers a variety of sushi rolls and traditional Japanese dishes such as the teriyaki chicken and the udon noodle soup.

No matter what type of cuisine you're in the mood for, San Jose has something to offer. From upscale restaurants to casual eateries, there's no shortage of options for a romantic night out in this vibrant city.

Napa Valley

Napa Valley is one of the most popular destinations in the Bay Area for wine lovers and foodies alike. Located just an hour north of San Francisco, this picturesque valley boasts over 400 wineries and some of the best restaurants in the country.

The Best Bay Area Restaurants for a Romantic Night Out

For those looking for a romantic night out in Napa Valley, there are a plethora of options to choose from. One of the most popular restaurants in the area is The French Laundry, which has been awarded three Michelin stars and is consistently ranked as one of the best restaurants in the world. The menu features French-inspired cuisine made with local and seasonal ingredients, and the wine list is extensive and carefully curated.

Another popular spot is The Restaurant at Meadowood, which has also been awarded three Michelin stars. The menu features contemporary American cuisine with a focus on local and sustainable ingredients, and the wine list features over 1,200 different labels.

For those looking for something a bit more casual, there are also plenty of options. Oenotri is a popular Italian restaurant that sources many of their ingredients from their own farm, and offers a wide selection of gluten-free options. The menu features house-made pastas, wood-fired pizzas, and a variety of meat and seafood dishes.

Another great option is Archetype, which features a California-inspired menu with a focus on fresh, seasonal ingredients. The restaurant offers a variety of gluten-free options, including gluten-free bread and pasta, and the menu changes frequently to reflect the changing seasons.

No matter what type of cuisine you're in the mood for, Napa Valley has something for everyone. From Michelin-starred restaurants to casual cafes, this beautiful valley is a food lover's paradise, and the perfect destination for a romantic night out.

Chapter 5: Tips for Planning a Romantic Night Out

Making Reservations

Making Reservations

When it comes to planning a romantic night out at one of the best Bay Area restaurants, making reservations is a must. With so many popular dining spots in the region, it's important to plan ahead and secure your spot at the table. Here are some tips for making reservations at Bay Area restaurants.

1. Plan Ahead

Many of the top restaurants in the Bay Area book up weeks or even months in advance, especially during peak dining times like weekends, holidays, and special occasions. To avoid disappointment, it's best to start planning your romantic night out at least a few weeks in advance. Check the restaurant's website or call ahead to find out their reservation policy and availability.

2. Be Flexible

The Best Bay Area Restaurants for a Romantic Night Out

If your preferred date or time is already booked, try to be flexible with your plans. Consider dining at a different time of day, such as a late lunch or early dinner, or on a less popular day of the week. You may also want to consider alternative dining options, such as outdoor seating or a private dining room.

3. Communicate Any Dietary Restrictions

If you or your partner has any dietary restrictions, such as gluten-free or vegetarian, make sure to communicate this to the restaurant when making your reservation. Many Bay Area restaurants are happy to accommodate special dietary needs, but they may need advance notice to prepare accordingly.

4. Confirm Your Reservation

A few days before your reservation, it's always a good idea to confirm your booking with the restaurant. This will ensure that there are no last-minute changes or misunderstandings that could impact your romantic night out.

By following these tips, you can ensure that your romantic night out at one of the best Bay Area restaurants is a success. Whether you're looking for a cozy bistro or a fine dining experience, the Bay Area is home to some of the most romantic restaurants in the country. So, start planning your perfect night out today!

Dress Code

The Best Bay Area Restaurants for a Romantic Night Out

When it comes to planning a romantic night out at a Bay Area restaurant, it's important to take note of the dress code. While some restaurants may have more relaxed attire requirements, others may have specific guidelines that must be followed in order to dine there. Understanding the dress code will ensure that you and your partner are appropriately dressed and comfortable throughout the evening.

For those looking for a more upscale dining experience, the dress code is likely to be more formal. Men may be required to wear a jacket and tie, while women may be expected to wear a dress or skirt. It's always a good idea to check the restaurant's website or call ahead to confirm the dress code before arriving. This will save you any embarrassment or discomfort if you are not dressed appropriately.

On the other hand, if you're looking for a more relaxed dining experience, there are plenty of options available in the Bay Area. Casual restaurants may have a more lenient dress code, allowing for comfortable clothing such as jeans and a nice blouse or shirt. However, it's still important to present yourself well and show respect for the restaurant and its staff.

If you have specific dietary needs, such as gluten-free, it's important to also consider this when choosing your attire. Many gluten-free restaurants may have a more casual dress code, but it's still important to dress appropriately. Comfortable and breathable clothing that allows for movement and flexibility will ensure that you can enjoy your meal without any discomfort.

The Best Bay Area Restaurants for a Romantic Night Out

Ultimately, the dress code should not deter you from enjoying a romantic night out at one of the Bay Area's best restaurants. Whether you prefer a more formal or casual dining experience, there are plenty of options available. Just remember to dress appropriately and be respectful of the restaurant's guidelines.

Transportation

Transportation is an important aspect of planning a romantic night out in the Bay Area. With the abundance of traffic and limited parking, it's important to consider your transportation options to ensure a stress-free and enjoyable evening.

One option is public transportation. The Bay Area has an extensive network of buses, trains, and ferries that can take you to your destination without the hassle of driving. BART, Muni, and Caltrain are popular options for getting around San Francisco, while the ferry system is a great way to explore the Bay Area's waterfront restaurants.

Another option is ride-sharing services such as Uber or Lyft. These services allow you to easily get to and from your destination without worrying about parking or navigating through traffic. Additionally, some restaurants offer discounts or promotions for ride-sharing users, so be sure to check with your selected restaurant before arriving.

The Best Bay Area Restaurants for a Romantic Night Out

For those who prefer to drive, consider carpooling with friends or using a car-sharing service such as Zipcar. This not only reduces the number of cars on the road but also allows you to split the cost of transportation with others.

Finally, for a truly romantic and unique experience, consider renting a limousine or private car. This allows you to sit back and relax while someone else handles the driving. Many limousine companies offer special packages for romantic nights out, including champagne, roses, and other romantic touches.

Regardless of your transportation choice, be sure to plan ahead and factor in travel time to ensure a stress-free and enjoyable evening at one of the Bay Area's best romantic restaurants. Whether you're following the Bay Area Restaurant Guide or the Gluten-Free Bay Area Restaurant Guide, transportation is key to a successful night out.

Preparing for Dietary Restrictions

Preparing for Dietary Restrictions

For those with dietary restrictions, dining out can be a daunting task. The good news is that many Bay Area restaurants are well-equipped to handle a variety of dietary needs, including gluten-free, vegetarian, and vegan options. Here are a few tips to help you prepare for your next night out:

1. Do Your Research

The Best Bay Area Restaurants for a Romantic Night Out

Before choosing a restaurant, do a little research to make sure they can accommodate your dietary needs. Many restaurants have menus available online, which can be helpful in determining if they have options that meet your restrictions. Additionally, websites like Yelp and OpenTable often have reviews and comments from diners with dietary restrictions, which can give you a better idea of how well the restaurant handles those needs.

2. Call Ahead

If you have a severe allergy or other dietary restriction, it's a good idea to call the restaurant ahead of time to let them know about your needs. This will give them time to prepare and ensure that they have options available for you.

3. Be Specific

When ordering, be clear and specific about your dietary needs. Don't assume that the server or chef knows what you mean by "gluten-free" or "vegan." Instead, ask questions and provide as much detail as possible about what you can and cannot eat.

4. Be Open-Minded

While it can be tempting to stick to familiar dishes that you know are safe for your dietary needs, don't be afraid to try something new. Many restaurants have creative and delicious options that are specifically designed for those with dietary restrictions.

5. Be Prepared to Pay More

Unfortunately, dining out with dietary restrictions can often be more expensive than ordering from the regular menu. This is because restaurants often have to use more expensive ingredients to accommodate specific needs. Be prepared to pay a little extra for these options.

By following these tips, you can enjoy a romantic night out at one of the Bay Area's best restaurants, even if you have dietary restrictions. Remember to do your research, be specific when ordering, and be open-minded about trying new dishes. With a little preparation, you can have a memorable dining experience that meets all of your dietary needs.

Chapter 6: Conclusion

Recap of Top Bay Area Romantic Restaurants

Recap of Top Bay Area Romantic Restaurants

The Bay Area is home to some of the most romantic restaurants in the country. From fine dining to casual eateries, the region offers a plethora of options for couples looking for a special night out. In this chapter, we will recap some of the best romantic restaurants in the Bay Area.

The Best Bay Area Restaurants for a Romantic Night Out

One of the top romantic restaurants in the Bay Area is Acquerello in San Francisco. This Italian fine-dining restaurant serves elegant dishes made with locally-sourced ingredients. The dimly-lit dining room with white tablecloths and soft music sets the perfect ambiance for a romantic evening.

Another great spot for a romantic dinner is the French-inspired restaurant, The Village Pub in Woodside. The cozy dining room with a fireplace and elegant décor creates a warm and inviting atmosphere. The menu features seasonal ingredients and a great selection of wine.

If you are looking for a more casual yet romantic setting, The Cliff House in San Francisco is a great option. The restaurant offers stunning views of the Pacific Ocean and serves classic American dishes. It is a perfect spot for a romantic sunset dinner.

For those who are gluten-free, there are many romantic restaurants in the Bay Area that cater to their dietary needs. One of the best is Pausa in San Mateo. This Italian restaurant offers an extensive gluten-free menu with delicious pasta dishes made with gluten-free flour.

If you are looking for a romantic brunch spot, Plow in San Francisco is a great option. The cozy restaurant serves farm-to-table dishes made with organic and locally-sourced ingredients. The rustic décor and warm atmosphere make it a perfect spot for a romantic breakfast or brunch.

The Best Bay Area Restaurants for a Romantic Night Out

In conclusion, the Bay Area offers a diverse range of romantic restaurants for couples to enjoy. From fine-dining to casual eateries, there is something for every taste and budget. Whether you are looking for a gluten-free option or a cozy spot for brunch, there is a restaurant in the Bay Area that will suit your needs.

Final Thoughts and Recommendations

Final Thoughts and Recommendations

As we come to the end of this guide, we hope that we have provided you with some valuable information on the best Bay Area restaurants for a romantic night out. We know that choosing the perfect restaurant can be a daunting task. However, with this guide at your disposal, you can rest easy knowing that you have access to some of the most romantic and delectable dining options in the region.

For our gluten-free readers, we have also provided a comprehensive guide to the best Bay Area restaurants that cater to your dietary needs. We understand how difficult it can be to find restaurants that offer gluten-free options that are not only safe but also delicious. Therefore, we hope that this guide has been helpful in narrowing down your options and giving you the confidence to dine out without worry.

Our final recommendation is to always make reservations in advance, especially for those special romantic occasions. Bay Area restaurants are popular and can get busy quickly, so it's essential to plan ahead to avoid disappointment.

The Best Bay Area Restaurants for a Romantic Night Out

Lastly, we encourage you to explore the Bay Area's diverse culinary scene and try out new restaurants. The region is home to some of the world's most innovative and exciting chefs, and there's always something new to discover. Whether you're in the mood for classic Italian cuisine, fresh seafood, or modern fusion dishes, the Bay Area has something for everyone.

In conclusion, we hope that this guide has been a valuable resource for our readers. We have enjoyed sharing our knowledge and experiences with you and wish you the best of luck in your future dining adventures. Bon Appétit!

www.ingramcontent.com/pod-product-compliance
Lightning Source LLC
Chambersburg PA
CBHW060033040426
42333CB00042B/2434